Behavioural Interventions to Eliminate Cardiovascular Diseases Without Surgery

Scientifically Proven Healthy Lifestyle For Heart Diseases Prevention And Care

by

Arnold Bridge M.D

I0504402

Dedication

For Christiana, jewel with a heart of gold!

<u>Acknowledgements</u>

My esteem regards to my colleagues for their unalloyed support during the preparation of this book.

Table of Contents

CHAPTER ONE

1.0 Cardiovascular Diseases: The Basics

There are increasing studies on care for the heart due to the prevalence of heart diseases. This text explores the fast, easy-to-understand guide to understanding the causes, diagnosis and symptoms of each type of heart disease with proven treatment. As advances are made daily in the research and treatment of heart disease, a new study posits that fat distribution across the body increases the risk of heart disease. Remarkably, heart disease can be treated with medication or surgery. Arrhythmia, Coronary heart disease, and Myocardial infarction are some examples of heart diseases. Coronary Heart Disease is the most common type of heart disease. The notorious Coronary Artery Disease is said to be America's No.1 killer, affecting more than 13 million Americans.

The condition that develops when a substance called plaque builds up in the walls of the arteries, narrowing the arteries and making it harder for blood to flow through is referred to as Atherosclerosis. The term "heart disease" is used interchangeably with the term "cardiovascular disease"; the latter, being a condition that involve narrowed or blocked blood vessels that can result in heart attack, chest pain (angina) or stroke.

With respect to treatment of heart diseases, quitting smoking and exercising regularly are helpful tips. Some notable diseases under the heart disease umbrella include blood vessel diseases, such as heart defects that originated from birth (congenital heart defects), heart rhythm problems (arrhythmias); coronary artery disease; among others.

As will be espoused, various noteworthy research on heart disease has affirmed the following:

-High-intensity interval exercise is beneficial to heart transplant patients.

-Risk of heart disease increase by 500 percent with baldness and gray hair in men

-Fat distribution across the body increases the risk of heart disease.

-To reduce this risk of heart disease, it is desirable to cut out cigarettes totally

-The risk of death appears higher for unmarried people, such as those who are widowed, divorced, separated, or never married than persons who are married.

1.1 Know Your Heart

The heart is a muscle with the size of the fist that pumps blood around the body and beats approximately 70 times a minute. Of note, the heart gets its own supply of blood from a network of blood vessels on the heart's surface known as- 'coronary arteries'. The process by which the heart operates in the body is known as- 'circulation'. When blood departs from the right side of the heart, it goes straight to the lungs where it picks up oxygen; thereafter, the oxygen-rich blood returns to the heart and is then pumped to the body's organs through a network of arteries. Afterwards, the blood returns to the heart through veins before being pumped back to the lungs again. This process is called circulation.

1.2 Statistics on Prevalence of Heart Disease

It has been confirmed by the Centers for Disease Control (CDC) that the leading cause of death in the United Kingdom, United States and Canada is heart disease. Further, it is the leading cause of death for several populations, including Caucasians, Hispanics, and African-Americans. Of note, heart disease doesn't discriminate. Almost half of Americans are at risk of one heart disease or the other since it is reported that one in every four deaths in the U.S. occurs as a result of heart disease. Mississippi is said to be the state with the highest rate of death from heart disease; followed by Oklahoma, Arkansas, Alabama, and Louisiana. The U.S. economy at large equally feels the impact.

CHAPTER TWO

2.0 Types of Heart Diseases

Overtime, a number of heart diseases have been identified due to their prevalence, as hereunder set out:

- **Hypertrophic Cardiomyopathy:** This is characterized by thickening of the walls of the heart. It is a peculiar genetic disorder in which the wall of the left ventricle thickens, thereby making it difficult for blood to be pumped out of the heart. There is 50 percent likelihood that parents with hypertrophic cardiomyopathy will pass the disorder to their children. Of note, it is the leading cause of sudden death in athletes.

- **Heart Muscle Disease (Cardiomyopathy):** This is a serious Heart muscle disease that usually affects the left ventricle. Dilated cardiomyopathy occurs when the heart chambers become dilated as a result of heart muscle weakness and cannot pump blood properly for various reasons such as inadequacy of the oxygen reaching the heart muscle, due to coronary artery disease. Dilated cardiomyopathy can appear at any age There could also be a minimal or restrictive Cardiomyopathy.

- **Arrhythmia or Irregular Heart Rhythm:** It results where the heart doesn't keep up a good beat or its regular rhythm that be too fast, too slowly, or too erratically or when the electrical impulses in the heart that coordinate the heartbeat do not work properly. It affects how well your heart works as the heart may not be able to pump enough blood to meet the body's needs. It is quite common, with the feel like a fluttering or a racing heart, but it is important to pay attention when they change too much or occur because of a damaged or weak heart since Arrhythmias can become fatal. There are various types of arrhythmias, viz:

a) Bradycardia: It entails a heart rate of less than 60 beats per minute. It occurs when the heart beats too slowly or the heart rate is too slow.

b) Premature Ventricular Contractions: This is exemplified by additional abnormal beats.

c) Fibrillation: It entails when the heartbeat is irregular. It's the most common kind of irregular heartbeat

d) Tachycardia: It entails a heart rate of more than 100 beats per minute. It occurs when the heart beats too fast or the heart rate is too fast.

- **Pericarditis:** The little sac that holds the heart is the pericardium and it can get infected. This infection is known as pericarditis or pericardial disease.

- **Pericardial Effusion:** The fluid around the heart can be caused by various types of infection/inflammation or cancer, kidney disease or heart surgery which impairs heart function.

- **Marfan Syndrome:** It is an inherited genetic defect that weakens connective tissues generally and those in the heart.

- **Heart valve problems:** Various forms of heart valve problems include-

a) Stenosis: It occurs when the valves do not open enough to allow the blood to flow through.

b) Prolapse: It occurs when the valve leaflets bulge back into the upper chamber as the valve between the left atrium and left ventricle does not fully close. This condition makes it difficult for the heart to pump blood from the right ventricle into the pulmonary artery because the pulmonary valve is too tight

c) Regurgitation: It is also known as mitral valve regurgitation, mitral insufficiency, or mitral incompetence. It occurs when the heart valves don't close properly and thus allows blood to flow back into the heart when it should leave.

People with this type of heart condition often feel tired and out of breath.

d) Heart Murmurs: This may be harmless but could equally result from blood flowing through a damaged or overworked heart valve. Otherwise, they may have resulted from blood flowing through healthy valves in a healthy heart hence not requiring treatment.

- **Sudden Cardiac Death:** The prevalence of this is quite alarming and it is reported to be the cause of half of all heart disease deaths and is a general term for some deformities of the heart that have been present since birth.

- **Congenital Heart Disease:** Remarkably this relates to the fact that some persons are born with heart disease. This is a general term for some deformities of the heart that have been present since birth. Examples include: Obstruction defects, Cyanotic heart disease, Septal defects, etc

- **Enlarged Heart (Cardiomegaly):** This usually caused by high blood pressure (hypertension) or coronary artery disease.

- **Stroke**: This condition is characterized by impairment of brain cells either temporary or permanent. Thus where the impaired cells repair themselves, previously impaired function improves. However, these cells may never replaced. Certain effects of stroke are permanent where many brain cells die resulting from starvation of oxygen. Two notable types of this condition are:

a) **Ischemic stroke:** It occurs when a blood vessel that feeds the brain gets blocked; this may have resulted from a blood clot. Herein, functions controlled by that part of the brain is diminished as the supply of blood to some parts of the brain is cut off, thereby causing the death of some brain cells.

b) **Hemorrhagic stroke:** It occurs when a blood vessel within the brain bursts. This could be as a result of high blood pressure

• **Heart failure:** This occurs when the heart failure occurs when though the heart has not stopped beating but the heart fails to pump blood around the body efficiently. It could be that the left or right side of the heart is affected. Heart failure can get worse if left untreated.

• **Myocardial Infarction/ Heart Attack/ Coronary Thrombosis:** This is characterized by an interruption of blood flow which damages or destroys part of the heart muscle resulting most times from a blood clot that develops in one of the coronary arteries. Of note, where the clot cuts off the blood flow completely, the part of the heart muscle supplied by that artery begins to die. This condition can also occur if an artery suddenly narrows.

- **Coronary Artery Disease:** Coronary heart disease (CHD), sometimes called Ischaemic Heart Disease is a major cause of death worldwide. Remarkably, it is the Coronary Arteries that supplies nutrients and oxygen to the heart muscle by circulating blood and can become diseased or damaged. The damage may result from plaque deposits that contain cholesterol. Plaque buildup narrows the coronary arteries, and this causes the heart to receive less oxygen and nutrients. Coronary heart disease is the term that describes what occurs when the heart's blood supply is blocked or interrupted by a build-up of fatty substances in the coronary arteries. The process by which the arteries are furred up with fatty deposits is known as atherosclerosis and the fatty deposits are called atheroma. Atherosclerosis can be caused by lifestyle factors and other conditions, such as:

✓ smoking

✓ high blood pressure (hypertension)

✓ diabetes

✓ high cholesterol

Main Symptoms of Coronary Heart Disease CHD

Though symptoms of CHD vary among individuals and some people may not have any before CHD is diagnosed, the main symptoms of Coronary Heart Disease CHD are:

-Angina (Chest Pain)

-Heart Attacks

-Heart Failure

Tests for Diagnosis of Coronary Heart Disease CHD

The tests that may be required in the diagnosis of CHD include:

❖　　A Treadmill Test

❖　　A Radionuclide Scan

❖　　A CT Scan

- ❖ An MRI Scan

- ❖ A Coronary Angiography

Treatment of Coronary Heart Disease CHD

Whilst Coronary Heart Disease is deadly and equally prevalent, one can reduce the risk of getting CHD by making some simple lifestyle changes. In the same vein, treatment can help manage the symptoms and reduce the chances of problems such as heart attacks. The treatment include:

➢ surgery

➢ lifestyle changes, such as regular exercise and stopping smoking

➢ medication

➢ angioplasty - using balloons and stents to treat narrow heart arteries

The notable desirable lifestyle changes to combat Coronary Heart Disease include:

- eating a healthy, balanced diet

- giving up smoking

- Keeping your heart healthy will also have other health benefits, such as helping reduce your risk of stroke and dementia.

- controlling blood cholesterol and sugar levels

- being physically active

CHAPTER THREE

3.0 Symptoms of Failing Heart

Overtime, it has been discovered that chest pain is common to many types of heart disease(known as angina, or angina pectoris- occurring when a part of the heart does not receive enough oxygen triggered by stressful events or physical exertion), however, as will be espoused different types of heart disease may result in a variety of symptoms. On the other hand, some heart conditions occur with no symptoms at all, especially in older adults and individuals with diabetes.

3.1 Heart Defects Symptoms

3.1.1 Heart Disease Symptoms for Congenital Heart Disease

This refers to a range of conditions. Whereas some heart defects are never diagnosed immediately after birth, in severe cases, symptoms can occur from birth whilst in other cases, the symptoms only get noticeable at a later age.

Symptoms of congenital heart defects that usually aren't immediately life-threatening include:

- Easily getting short of breath

- Easily getting exhausted during work

- Swelling in the hands, ankles or feet

Symptoms of congenital heart defects in children could include:

- Shortness of breath during feedings

- Pale gray or blue skin color

- Swelling in the abdomen, legs, or around the eyes

Common symptoms of congenital heart defects generally are:

- Breathlessness

- Chest pain

- Clubbed fingernails

- Unusual fatigue

- Fast heartbeat and breathing

- Blue-tinged skin

- Sweating

- Swelling of the extremities

- Irregular heart rhythm

3.1.2 Heart Disease Symptoms for Abnormal Heartbeats (Heart Arrhythmias)

Arrhythmias refers to an abnormal heartbeat. Your heart may beat too quickly, too slowly or irregularly. Heart arrhythmia symptoms can include:

- Slow Heartbeat (Bradycardia)

- Fainting Spells

- Slow Pulse

- Racing Heartbeat (Tachycardia)

- Chest Pain Or Discomfort

- Fluttering Chest

- Shortness Of Breath

- Lightheadedness

- Dizziness

- Fainting (Syncope) Or Near Fainting

3.1.3 Symptoms of Heart Disease In Blood Vessels (Atherosclerotic Disease)

Ordinarily, heart disease in blood vessels (atherosclerotic disease) reduces blood supply to extremities, but the symptoms of heart disease in the blood vessel may be different for men and women. For instance, whereas men are more likely to have chest pain; women are more likely to have shortness of breath, nausea and extreme fatigue. It can sometimes be diagnosed early with regular evaluations.

Symptoms of atherosclerosis include:

- Chest Tightness

- Numbness, Especially In The Limbs

- Shortness Of Breath

- Coldness, Especially In The Limbs

- Chest Pain

- Chest Pressure

- Pain In The Neck, Jaw, Throat, Upper Abdomen Or Back

- Weakness In Your Legs And Arms

- Chest Discomfort (Angina)

3.1.4 Heart Disease Symptoms for Weak Heart Muscle (Dilated Cardiomyopathy)

Cardiomyopathy ordinarily results in the muscles of the heart growing larger and turning rigid or weak. Symptoms include:

- Dizziness

- Bloating

- Shortness of breath

- Swelling of the legs, ankles and feet

- Fatigue

- Breathlessness with exertion or at rest

- Irregular heartbeats

- Lightheadedness and fainting

3.1.5 Heart Disease Symptoms for Heart Infections

The term- heart infection may be used to describe conditions such as endocarditis or myocarditis and it affects the inner membrane that separates the chambers and valves of the heart. Symptoms of a heart infection include:

- Skin rashes or unusual spots

- Fever

- Shortness of breath

- Weakness or fatigue

- Swelling in your legs or abdomen

- Changes in your heart rhythm

- Dry or persistent cough

3.1.6 Heart Disease Symptoms for Coronary Artery Disease (CAD)

Coronary Artery Disease is quite prevalent with the following symptoms:

- Nausea

- Chest pain

- Feelings of indigestion

- Feeling of pressure in the chest

- Shortness of breath

3.1.7 Heart Disease Symptoms for Valvular Heart Disease

Valves of the heart (the aortic, mitral, pulmonary and tricuspid valves) may be damaged by a number of conditions. The said conditions could lead to narrowing (stenosis), leaking (regurgitation or insufficiency) or improper closing (prolapse).

The symptoms of valvular heart disease include:

- Fatigue

- Swollen feet or ankles

- Shortness of breath

- Fainting

- Irregular heartbeat

- Chest pain

.

CHAPTER FOUR

4.0 Causes of Heart Disease

Generally, heart disease is caused by a number of factors such as damage to the coronary arteries, damage to part of the heart, or a poor supply of nutrients and oxygen to the organ.

Though some types of heart disease, such as hypertrophic cardiomyopathy are genetic, a number of lifestyle choices can increase the risk of heart disease.

4.1 Are You At Risk?

Whereas some risk factors for heart disease are controllable(for example- smoking), others are not(such as family history, ethnicity, sex, age etc).

Flowing from the above, some notable risk factors for heart disease include:

➢ Family history

➢ Smoking

- Certain chemotherapy drugs and radiation therapy for cancer.

- High blood pressure.

- Obesity

- Age

- Sex

- Poor diet

- Physical inactivity

- Stress

- High blood cholesterol levels

- Diabetes

- Poor hygiene

The aforelisted risk factors greatly increases the risk of heart disease. Save for genetically induced heart related diseases, poor lifestyle habits is a major cause of heart diseases. Hence, healthy diet, regular exercise, cholesterol-lowering drugs, and lifesaving surgeries are helpful to avoid a heart attack. Though Heart disease is said to be chronic a host of medications can control it.

Complications of heart disease include:

- ❖ Heart failure

- ❖ Peripheral artery disease

- ❖ Sudden cardiac arrest

- ❖ Heart attack

- ❖ Stroke

- ❖ Aneurysm

Most heart attacks are the end result of coronary heart disease, a condition that clogs coronary arteries with fatty, calcified plaques. The causes of heart disease vary by type of heart disease. Hence, each category of heart disease is caused by a unique factor.

4.2 Causes of Cardiovascular Disease

Cardiovascular disease is characterized by a buildup of fatty plaques in the arteries that inhibit blood flow through the arteries to organs and tissues. Other causes are- unhealthy diet, being overweight, lack of exercise, and smoking. Atherosclerosis is the most common cause of cardiovascular disease

4.3 Causes of Heart Arrhythmia

Common causes of abnormal heart rhythms (arrhythmias) include:

- stress and anxiety

- existing heart damage or disease

- diabetes

- Smoking

- heart defects, including congenital heart defects

- medications, supplements, and herbal remedies

- high blood pressure (hypertension)

- excessive alcohol or caffeine use

- substance use disorders

4.4 Causes of Congenital Heart Defects

Some medical conditions, medications and genes can cause heart defects. It usually develop while a baby is in the womb. The heart's structure can change as you age. Heart defects can develop as the heart develop.

4.5 Causes of Cardiomyopathy

Since various types of cardiomyopathy exist, the cause of cardiomyopathy, a thickening or enlarging of the heart muscle, may depend on the type

4.6 Dilated Cardiomyopathy

This could result from reduced blood flow to the heart (ischemic heart disease) arising from damage after a heart attack, infections, toxins and certain drugs or inherited.

- **Hypertrophic cardiomyopathy**: This could result from high blood pressure or aging or inherited.

- **Restrictive cardiomyopathy**: This could result from diseases, such as connective tissue disorders, excessive iron buildup in your body (hemochromatosis), the buildup of abnormal proteins (amyloidosis) or by some cancer treatments.

4.7 Causes of Heart Infection

Bacteria, parasites, and viruses are the most common causes of heart infection.

4.8 Causes of Valvular Heart Disease

Whilst one may be born with valvular disease, it is equally possible for the valves to be damaged by conditions such as: Rheumatic fever, Infections or Connective tissue disorders.

CHAPTER FIVE

5.0 Prevention, Diagnosis And Treatment of Heart Disease

Whereas some types of heart disease, such as those that are present from birth, cannot be prevented, others can be prevented. This chapter focuses on how to deal with heart disease risk factors so you can have the best chance at avoiding heart disease. The following helps improve overall health and greatly reduce the chances of heart complications:

- Reduce and manage stress

-Having a balanced diet: Taking Heart-Healthy Diet helps. The fats in diet should be unsaturated. It is equally desireable to have to low-fat, high-fiber foods and stick with five portions of fresh fruit and vegetables each day. Increased intake of whole grains, reduced intake of salt and sugar in diet are helpful tips too.

-Regular exercise: This will help to strengthen the heart and circulatory system, reduce cholesterol, and maintain blood pressure.

-Control all conditions that affect heart health as a complication, such as high blood pressure or diabetes.

-Lower Your Cholesterol: Healthy body weight is advised.

-Exercise for Heart Disease Prevention

-Quit Smoking: Smoking is a major risk factor for heart and cardiovascular conditions.

-Alcohol and Heart Disease: Reduce the intake of alcohol.

5.1 Diagnosis of Heart Disease

Several types of tests and evaluations may be required to make a heart disease diagnosis. Some of these are hereunder set out-

5.1.1 Physical Exams And Blood Tests

overstated. Upon receiving a heart disease diagnosis, a detailed list of everyday habits to bear in mind includes:

-seeing the doctor regularly

- exercise routine

-medications

- diet

- family history of heart disease or stroke

-history of high blood pressure or diabetes

-any symptoms such as a racing heart, dizziness, or lack of energy

5.3 Is There A Cure For Heart Disease?

Heart disease usually requires a lifetime of treatment and careful monitoring. A good number of the symptoms of heart disease can be relieved with medications, procedures, and lifestyle changes, albeit, where these do not yield the required result, coronary intervention or bypass surgery might be resorted to. As a starting point, an attempt is made to treat the heart condition using medications, but where this is not yielding the desired result, surgical options are available. Treatment for heart disease must factor in the type of heart disease. Basically, treatment for heart disease falls into three broad main categories:

❖ Lifestyle changes

Having a healthy lifestyle goes a long way in treating any heart condition and prevent same from getting worse. Regular exercise, reduced alcohol consumption, low-sodium, low-fat diet, diet rich in fruits and vegetables and quitting tobacco.

❖ Medications

A medication may be necessary to treat certain types of heart disease. Your doctor can prescribe a medication can be prescribed as either a cure or to control heart disease or to slow down or stop the risk for complications. Drug prescriptions is determined by the type of heart disease in question. The main medications in use are:

-Beta-blockers, for treating heart attack, heart failure, and high blood pressure

-Angiotensin-converting enzyme (ace) inhibitors, for heart failure and high blood pressure

-Statins, for lowering cholesterol

-Aspirin, clopidogrel, and warfarin, for preventing blood clots

❖ Surgery Or Invasive Procedures

To prevent worsening symptoms in certain cases of heart disease surgery or a medical procedure is necessary to treat the condition. However, the procedure for the surgery to be adopted depends on on the type of heart disease and the extent of damage. The most common surgeries include:

- Angioplasty

- Pacemakers or electronic machines

- Heart transplants

- Coronary artery bypass surgery

- Curgery to repair or replace faulty heart valves

CHAPTER SIX

6.0 Feeding The Heart

Deaths resulting from heart disease is No. 1 killer of Americans. There is proven evidence of a nexus between diet and heart disease as some food influence blood pressure, triglycerides, cholesterol levels and inflammation. The term- GIGO (Garbage In Garbage Out) as applicable in computer parlance aptly captures the resultant effect of bad diet in humans. To avoid chronic heart diseases such as- Congestive heart failure (CHF), some diets are recommended to keep the heart in good shape. Preventing heart attacks entails not simply avoidance of unhealthy food, but equally having a healthy diet. Hence eating food in their natural form is highly recommended for the heart as well as waistline. Whereas for Congestive heart failure (CHF) which is attributable to extra fluid buildup affecting the heart's ability to pump blood, dietary changes to reduce sodium consumption and restricting fluid intake to reduce extra fluid is recommended. If you have congestive heart failure, follow these nutrition tips:

6.1 Nutrition Tips for Congestive Heart Failure

There are ways to help manage congestive heart failure with eating plan. Checking food labels, and limiting salt and sodium is desirable and this can be done in certain ways. Too much sodium can cause fluid retention. A low-salt diet helps keep high blood pressure and swelling under control. It can also make breathing easier if you have heart failure. Limiting salt and sodium can be done without sacrificing flavor through-

1. Swap salt for the following:

   a. Dill

   b. tarragon

   c. oregano

   d. basil

e. thyme

f. thyme

2. Be on the lookout for food containing high levels of sodium

3. Do away with consumption of prepackaged food or processed foods in cans or boxes

4. Study food labels

5. Notify the cook, chef or waiter of your preference early enough

6. Keeping track of body weight helps to know how the body is filtering fluid

7. Take fruits high in water and sodium-free such as watermelon

8. Distribute daily fluid consumption at intervals

9. Do away with salt shaker on the dining table

10. Resort to alternative thirst quenchers

11. When eating out, ensure compliance with your diet preference

11. Limit intake of cheese that are high in sodium

12. Eat fresh meats, chicken, and fish.

13. Recognize menu terms that may indicate a high sodium content

6.2 Nutrition Tips For Fat And Cholesterol Related Heart Problems

Fat and Cholesterol

The following tips are useful to replace a diet high in saturated fat and cholesterol which fuels heart problems:

a. Use canola oil or olive oil instead of solid fats when cooking.

b. Do away with consumption of red meat and replace with fish

c. Do away with consumption of fried food, and replace with boiled or steam foods

d. Take fat-free milk and dairy products

e. Limit added fats

f. Remove the skin from poultry before cooking

6.3 Heart Friendly Food

a. Oatmeal soaks up the cholesterol so it is eliminated from the body and not absorbed into the bloodstream due to its richness in soluble fiber, hence good for the body, likewise whole grains such as bread, pasta and grits.

b. Dark chocolate, ie. chocolate made up of at least 60-70% cocoa may help blood pressure, clotting, and inflammation.

c. Citrus fruits are equally beneficial

d. Avocado are rich in the monounsaturated fats that may lower heart disease risk factors, such as cholesterol

e. Pomegranates contain health-promoting compounds

f. Green tea reduces risk of cardiovascular disease and heart disease

g. Garlic has been used as a natural remedy to treat a variety of ailments and can even help improve heart health

h. Olive oil lowers the risk of heart disease

i. Tomatoes are high in heart-healthy potassium as well.

j. Coffee could equally lower the risk of cardiovascular disease and stroke

k. Almonds, walnuts, pistachios, peanuts and macadamia nuts are rich in fiber.

l. Soy products are a good way to add protein to diet without unhealthy fats and cholesterol

m.   Potatoes can be good for your heart since they are rich in potassium

n. Fatty fish such as sardines and mackerel and likewise salmon are heart friendly meals since they are rich in omega-3 fatty acids, proven to lower the risk of rhythmia (irregular heart beat) and atherosclerosis (plaque build-up in the arteries) and decrease triglycerides.

6.4 Heart Friendly Fruits

a) Crisp, fresh broccoli florets dipped in hummus

b) Berries such as blue berries and strawberries lower risk of heart attack

c) Oranges

d) Cantaloupes

e) Yellow and orange veggies such as carrots, sweet potatoes, red peppers and acorn squash help the heart. Leafy green vegetables are also well-known for their wealth of vitamins, minerals and antioxidants

f) Papaya

g) Tomatoes